Also by Anthea Peries

Addictions

Quit Gambling: How To Overcome Your Betting Addiction Symptoms Causes Proven Treatment Recovery

Shopping Addiction: Overcome Excessive Buying. Quit Impulse Purchasing, Save Money And Avoid Debt

Cancer and Chemotherapy

Coping with Cancer & Chemotherapy Treatment: What You Need to Know to Get Through Chemo Sessions

Coping with Cancer: How Can You Help Someone with Cancer, Dealing with Cancer Family Member, Facing Cancer Alone, Dealing with Terminal Cancer Diagnosis, Chemotherapy Treatment & Recovery

Chemotherapy Survival Guide: Coping with Cancer & Chemotherapy Treatment Side Effects

Chemotherapy Chemo Side Effects And The Holistic Approach: Alternative, Complementary And Supplementary Proven Treatments Guide For Cancer Patients

Eating Disorders
Food Cravings: Simple Strategies to Help Deal with Craving for Sugar & Junk Food
Sugar Cravings: How to Stop Sugar Addiction & Lose Weight
The Immune System, Autoimmune Diseases & Inflammatory Conditions: Improve Immunity, Eating Disorders & Eating for Health
Food Addiction: Overcome Sugar Bingeing, Overeating on Junk Food & Night Eating Syndrome
Food Addiction: Overcoming your Addiction to Sugar, Junk Food, and Binge Eating
Food Addiction: Why You Eat to Fall Asleep and How to Overcome Night Eating Syndrome
Overcome Food Addiction: How to Overcome Food Addiction, Binge Eating and Food Cravings
Healthy Gut: Transform Your Health from the Inside Out, for a Healthy You
Emotional Eating: Stop Emotional Eating & Develop Intuitive Eating Habits to Keep Your Weight Down
Emotional Eating: Overcoming Emotional Eating, Food Addiction and Binge Eating for Good
Eating At Night Time: Sleep Disorders, Health and Hunger Pangs: Tips On What You Can Do About It
Addiction To Food: Proven Help For Overcoming Binge Eating Compulsion And Dependence

Food Addiction

Overcoming Food Addiction to Sugar, Junk Food. Stop Binge Eating and Bad Emotional Eating Habits

Food Addiction: Overcoming Emotional Eating, Binge Eating and Night Eating Syndrome

Weight Loss Without Dieting: 21 Easy Ways To Lose Weight Naturally

Grief, Bereavement, Death, Loss

Coping with Loss & Dealing with Grief: Surviving Bereavement, Healing & Recovery After the Death of a Loved One

How to Plan a Funeral

Coping With Grief And Heartache Of Losing A Pet: Loss Of A Beloved Furry Companion: Easing The Pain For Those Affected By Animal Bereavement

Grieving The Loss Of Your Baby: Coping With The Devastation Shock And Heartbreak Of Losing A Child Through Miscarriage, Still Birth

Seeking Salvation, Secure In Belief: How To Get Sure-Fire Saved By Grace Through Faith, Rapture Ready And Heaven Bound

Loss And Grief: Treatment And Discovery Understanding Bereavement, Moving On From Heartbreak And Despair To Recovery

Health Fitness

How To Avoid Colds and Flu Everyday Tips to Prevent or Lessen The Impact of Viruses During Winter Season

Quark Cheese
50 More Ways to Use Quark Low-fat Soft Cheese: The Natural Alternative When Cooking Classic Meals
Quark Cheese Recipes: 21 Delicious Breakfast Smoothie Ideas Using Quark Cheese
30 Healthy Ways to Use Quark Low-fat Soft Cheese

Quit Alcohol
How To Stop Drinking Alcohol: Coping With Alcoholism, Signs, Symptoms, Proven Treatment And Recovery

Relationships
The Grief Of Getting Over A Relationship Breakup: How To Accept Breaking Up With Your Ex | Advice And Tips To Move On

Sleep Disorders
Sleep Better at Night and Cure Insomnia Especially When Stressed

Standalone

Family Style Asian Cookbook: Authentic Eurasian Recipes: Traditional Anglo-Burmese & Anglo-Indian

Coping with Loss and Dealing with Grief: The Stages of Grief and 20 Simple Ways on How to Get Through the Bad Days

Coping With Grief Of A Loved One After A Suicide: Grieving The Devastation And Loss Of Someone Who Took Their Own Life. How Long Does The Heartache Last?

When A Person Goes Missing And Cannot Be Found: Coping With The Grief And Devastation, Without Losing Hope, Of When An Adult Or Child Disappears

Menopause For Women: Signs Symptoms And Treatments A Simple Guide

Remembering Me: Discover Your Memory Proven Ways To Expand & Increase It As You Get Older

Boredom: How To Overcome Feeling Bored Discover Over 100 Proven Ways To Beat Apathy

Table of Contents

Introduction 3

The Process Of Chemotherapy Treatment 9

Stage Of Cancer Chemotherapy Is Used 13

Chemotherapy Pain Management 19

After Cancer Diagnosis 21

Amount Of Chemo Rounds 23

Chemotherapy Treatment And Your Personality 27

Chemo Brain 31

Chemotherapy Equipment Used 37

Stage 1 Cancer And Chemotherapy 39

The Success Rate Of Chemotherapy 41

What You Should Not Do During Chemotherapy 43

Boosting Your Immune System During Chemotherapy 45

Food For Chemotherapy And Radiation Therapy Cancer Treatment In General 53

Is Chemotherapy Working 57

The Pros And Cons Of Chemotherapy Treatment 59

Chemotherapy And Long-Term Damage 63

Foods That Help Shrink Tumours 65

Researching Complementary and Alternative therapies 69

Combining Supplementing Treatment With Alternative Therapies 75

Alternative Complementary Cancer Treatments 81

Is Chemotherapy Safe? 93

Questions To Ask Before Chemotherapy Treatment 95

God And Chemotherapy Treatment. 99

About The Author 105

Other Books By This Author 107

CHEMOTHERAPY

CHEMO SIDE EFFECTS

AND THE HOLISTIC APPROACH

Alternative, Complementary And Supplementary Proven Treatments Guide

For Cancer Patients

Anthea Peries

Copyright © 2021 by Anthea Peries

All rights reserved.

No part of this book may be reproduced without the copyright owner's written permission, except for the use of limited quotations for book reviews.

Disclaimer This book is not intended as a substitute for the medical oncology advice of physicians and other medical professionals or experts. It is not a medical book. At the time it was written, the information contained in this book may have changed. Please seek medical advice from your doctor or oncologist.

Introduction

Are you sure about your decision to have chemotherapy treatment?

If you are not sure, it may be a good idea to see a doctor who has experience treating cancer patients before making any decision. Although chemotherapy is one of our most successful treatments, it is also one of our most brutal.

Your body experiences an extreme change during the treatment process, and the new normal can last for up to two years. The side effects of chemotherapy are not always easy to accept, but they become an inevitable part of your life.

That being said, there are good and bad things about chemotherapy, so it is good to weigh the positives of chemotherapy treatment against the negatives.

Does your doctor have experience with treating cancer patients?

If you have any questions or concerns about facing chemotherapy, don't hesitate to ask.

Can you lead an everyday life after chemotherapy?

Yes. People with cancer go back to normal activities after chemotherapy—including work, school and sports. However, some people feel tired or get a little more tired than usual from the treatments.

So you might be tired after your treatments or have a headache or low blood counts. In addition, some side effects of chemotherapy can last for several weeks or longer after treatment ends, including side effects to the heart, lungs, stomach and bladder. Also, some loss of hair may be permanent.

Chemotherapy is mainly given to adults and older children. When cancer is treated in babies, it is called pediatric or pediatric oncology.

What does chemotherapy treat?

If the treatment helps shrink a tumour, it may mean that you can have surgery. Surgery may be used to remove only the part of cancer that spread or whole cancer. If you have had surgery for cancer, you will get chemotherapy afterwards to kill any cancer cells that may remain in your body. If a tumour does not shrink with chemotherapy or comes back after surgery, chemotherapy will not be helpful. But sometimes, doctors use chemotherapy just to relieve symptoms and make the patient feel better.

What types of cancer are treated with chemotherapy?

Many different types of cancer are treated with chemotherapy. Some common cancers treated with chemotherapy include lung cancer, breast cancer, colorectal cancer and prostate cancer.

Chemotherapy is used If the tumour cells cannot be removed by surgery or high levels of specific proteins in the blood that moves between tissues.

As mentioned above, some people getting treatment for other cancers will also get chemotherapy after their tumours have been removed to kill any remaining cancer cells.

Which chemotherapy drugs can be given by mouth?

For other cancers, it is not possible to remove the tumour surgically.

For some cancers, the main goal of treatment is to relieve symptoms. So, the first step in cancer treatment is often to treat the symptoms.

ChemoActive works differently from other cancer treatments because it uses natural plant extracts to reduce pain and nausea. ChemoActive can be used with or without surgery; however, ChemoActive has not been tested for long-term use in people with cancer.

What is ChemoActive?

We will discuss this later in the combining and supplementing treatment section of this book.

This book answers common questions and more. It also addresses complementary, supplementary and alternative treatments to consider, with your chemotherapy treatment. The book can be read sequentially or by the section.

I hope you find it of valuable and the information is helpful when considering your treatment. Your oncology doctor will discuss your options with you but it makes matters easier for you to be fairly knowledgeable about this subject. Cancer treatment is not just a one-drug solution. The more choices, the better.

The Process Of Chemotherapy Treatment

What happens with chemotherapy treatment?

Chemotherapy is a cancer treatment that uses medications to destroy cancer cells in the body. It's most often used to kill cancer cells that have spread beyond the original tumour site or are otherwise difficult to treat. Chemotherapy can be given intravenously through a needle inserted into one of the large veins near the heart, by mouth, or applied directly to an external surface such as skin, muscles, or mucous membranes.

Chemotherapy drugs enter and travel through the bloodstream throughout your entire body. The drugs can reach cancer cells by entering the bloodstream and seeping out of the capillaries near the cancer cells.

When used to treat solid tumours, chemotherapy drugs are sometimes injected into or near a tumour. Doctors might advise surgical removal of the primary tumour before starting treatment with chemotherapy. This is done to limit the amount of cancer that could potentially spread if chemotherapy isn't used or treatment fails.

Another method is injecting a targeted drug directly into a solid tumour while simultaneously surrounding it with normal fluid (also called embolization), which prevents the spread of the drug beyond the initial tumour site. In addition, some medications are injected directly into tumours when they cannot be removed physically or surgically.

Researchers are developing additional methods for administering chemotherapy drugs, such as nanoparticle-based delivery. This is a newer area of research that involves the use of tiny particles that can carry drugs directly to the cancerous cells.

It's still not certain how chemotherapy affects cancer or what kind of "mechanism" it has, but it's known that the effect of chemotherapy can kill some cancer cells. In addition, some drugs used in chemotherapy have been shown to slow the growth of tumour cells and even promote the death of susceptible cancer cells. Chemotherapy may also affect normal or healthy tissue in your body.

Types of chemotherapy and drugs used in chemotherapy are listed below.

Chemotherapy is categorized by type of anti-cancer drug. The type of chemotherapy is determined by the cancer type or stage, nature of the patient's tumour, and overall health status.

A common form of chemotherapy is called "chemotherapy" or "antitumor treatment". It's a group of drugs used together for cancer treatments administered intravenously (by injection into a vein) or given orally. These drugs kill cancer cells by damaging DNA molecules.

Some chemotherapy treatments are given in combination with radiation therapy, surgery, or other anti-cancer therapies to prevent or slow the growth of cancer cells that haven't yet spread.

Chemotherapy is also used to treat cancers that have spread to other parts of the body, such as when a person has liver cancer and cannot remove the tumour altogether.

Chemotherapy can be used alone or in combination with another type of therapeutic care to treat cancers such as *lymphoma, sarcoma, and leukaemia*. They attack rapidly dividing cells, making them no longer able to divide.

Chemotherapy is also used to treat other types of cancers such as gastrointestinal (G), breast, prostate, skin, and lung cancers.

Chemotherapy has been used for cancer treatment since the 1950s. The term "chemotherapy" was first used in the 1950s by Elie Metchnikoff of the Pasteur Institute in Paris when he studied ageing and suggested that "living organisms were exposed to factors that destroy them". The term was first used in a paper dated April 27, 1955. Since then, many types of cancer have been treated with chemotherapy drugs, and hundreds of millions of people have received anti-cancer treatment.

For the most common types of childhood cancers, acute lymphoblastic leukaemia in children and Hodgkin's disease in adolescents, chemotherapy is the primary method for managing these diseases.

Chemotherapy has been used to treat various forms of cancer for over 50 years. At first, it was used only when other treatments had failed. Now it's often used as the first treatment after surgery. Chemotherapy may also be used when a tumour is found early but hasn't spread widely or when tumours have spread throughout the body but not widely metastasized (spread).

Despite advances in surgical techniques and drug development - including immunotherapy - chemotherapy remains an important treatment option for all types of cancer.

Stage Of Cancer Chemotherapy Is Used

Chemotherapy is used as a second-line treatment. If it is felt that the patient's cancer has progressed to a stage where the benefits of surgery would not be worthwhile and if there are no apparent side-effects of the chemotherapy, then chemotherapy can be given. The stage of cancer is assessed by biopsy.

What type of chemotherapy does your oncologist use?

What is the process of chemotherapy treatment?

It depends on the type of tumour; often, one can get advice from their oncologist.

Examples of the kinds of chemotherapy include:

The process of chemotherapy treatment can be broken down into different steps. As a result, the dosage may differ in each step.

The first stage exercises the healthy cells in the body to fight back against cancer within them. The healthy cells will respond to this by getting stronger and multiplying. This is called "cytostatic conditioning". You will feel unwell during this stage because your body is being affected by it. Your doctor/nurse will tell you what to expect. The types of chemotherapy used during this stage are "cytopharm" and "paclitaxel".

How much chemotherapy will you have?

You will be given a tablet once every 3-4 days. It is taken with food to minimize stomach upset. The dosage is:

When and how often should my oncologist see me?

Your oncologist sees you every 2-3 weeks if you wish. Your doctor must attend the appointment to keep up to date with your treatment.

What is the maintenance stage?

During the maintenance stage, you have three doses of chemotherapy once every 3-4 weeks. This is called "granisetron" and "5-fluorouracil".

The maintenance dose depends on your body's tolerance to drugs. It can be anywhere from 1 to 10 tablets per dose. The reason for this is that cancer cells can return if they are not wiped out entirely. The maintenance stage aims to prevent this from happening. Therefore, it seeks to keep cancer cells at a low level in the blood circulation system.

How long will you have chemotherapy?

The duration that someone will have chemotherapy is based on their clinical condition/history. It is essential that someone completes chemotherapy as the role of chemotherapy is to prevent cancer from coming back. It is recommended that you see your oncologist once every 2-3 weeks during this period.

What are the side effects, and what are the signs of a reaction?

The side effects vary depending on which drug(s) you have been given. However, some common side effects include:

- *Itching*
- *redness and burning at the injection site.*
- *Vomiting, diarrhoea, flu-like symptoms, fatigue and generally "all over body" aches and pains.*

What can I do at home to help with my chemotherapy treatment?

Your oncologist will tell you what you can do at home. However, certain things can be done to ease the side effects. Some of these include:

The above information is not about the type of cancer. Instead, it's about the type of chemotherapy used as a second-line treatment.

It is essential that someone is aware of this information and knows what they are dealing with to ask any questions or request clarification from their oncologist or nurse.

See: Some U.K. oncologists have stated that knowledge of chemotherapy is not helpful for the effective treatment of cancer. They argue that "it is a dead-end". The reason is that chemotherapy aims to kill the cells, including remaining cancer cells. So, without blood vessels and with no immune system, what can you do?

It does not matter if you know about specific side effects from your oncologist or nurse, as long as they tell you the truth. The important thing is to get on with the treatments and let them do their job to treat/prevent cancer—letting them know what's happening will help.

For example: Letting your nurse know if you are not eating to help you; let your oncologist know if you are feeling unwell or tired, so they can help you feel better as quickly as possible.

When someone is told their cancer is incurable, it is essential to get a second opinion. Alternatively, it might be helpful to try different treatments and have more surgery.

It might be possible that all the cancer cells have not been taken out, especially if someone has had surgery in the last few years. So, getting another scan or biopsy will be helpful.

Chemotherapy Pain Management

Each person's body reacts differently to chemotherapy. You may or may not have painful side effects. If you experience pain or discomfort during treatment, let your healthcare team know right away. They will be able to help you manage your discomfort.

Where does it hurt?

Pain can occur anywhere in the body, but it is most often felt:

mouth, throat, bladder, bone marrow, abdomen, and skin.

Pain that occurs in other areas is not cancer.

What can I expect during chemo?

During treatment, you may have nausea or vomiting when your body does not want to take in any food or liquid. You may also feel tired and weak.

In addition, you may have bowel symptoms such as pain or discomfort or changes in bowel movements. Your doctor will give you instructions about managing the pain and discomfort to get through treatment.

You may need to bring a notebook, pen and other items with you to your chemotherapy treatment.

The following are some things that you can do while getting chemotherapy that will help you manage pain and discomfort, feel well and keep up your strength:

- *Have a listen to music or audiobooks.*
- *Bring magazines or books.*
- *Play games on a cell phone or tablet (as long as the device is waterproof).*
- *Get together with family and friends for lunch.*
- *Take a short nap.*
- *Do some stretching or yoga to help your body relax.*
- *Drink plenty of fluids throughout the day.*

Some people find it helpful to have someone close by during treatment to talk with about their experience. This may be a friend, family member, or caregiver. You may also want to bring something special such as music, pictures or cards to keep you company.

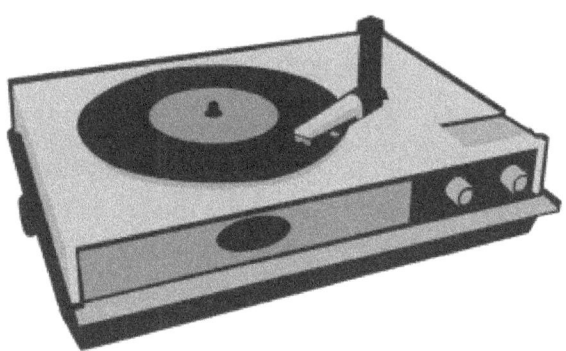

After Cancer Diagnosis

Chemotherapy may be recommended as part of your cancer treatment. This is the use of medicines to kill cancer cells and stop them from growing.

Your doctor will explain the kind of chemotherapy you might have, how long it will last, and whether it's likely to work. You also need to decide if you'll have more than one kind of treatment at a time. You must understand what is involved in your treatment.

Chemotherapy is usually given in cycles. A cycle is a period of chemotherapy treatment, followed by another period of rest. Each cycle is usually 28 days long. The length of each cycle will be worked out with you, based on your type and stage of cancer and other medical factors.

You may have more than one treatment in each cycle. The number of treatments you'll need depends on your type and stage of cancer, how well the cancers respond to treatment, and whether any other health problems could make you more vulnerable to chemotherapy.

The doctors who treat you should discuss how the chemotherapy will affect your quality of life and its chance to cure cancer or control its growth.

Amount Of Chemo Rounds

The number of rounds of chemo treatment varies. Sometimes it is 3 or 4 while sometimes more.

How many days a month is a chemotherapy?

Chemotherapy can last as long as six weeks, but most people will do it a week at a time. We count by weeks, but you will usually have 2–3 days off between treatments.

What do I do if I am having chemotherapy?

You will be asked to come in and see your nurse at least two times each week for your treatment. Your nurse will ask you how you feel so that the treatment can be adjusted if needed (which happens frequently). For example, you may feel sick to your stomach or have diarrhoea. You may also experience heartburn, fatigue, nausea, and vomiting. Your nurse will give you treatment for any symptoms you have.

When the chemo is finished, your nurse will see you ensure no problems related to the treatments. If you have a fever and start to feel dizzy or weak, your nurse can check the area where the chemo was given not to spread any further.

Do I need to eat or drink anything while I am having chemo?

There is no need for food or drink while under treatment. You can eat and drink as usual after this is over.

What is the difference between chemo and radiation?

Chemotherapy is given continuously, with the primary goal being to kill cancer cells. However, radiation kills only the cancer cells that are exposed to it.

Does chemo hurt?

Chemotherapy can cause some pain, but it is generally tolerable. The most common side effect of chemotherapy depends on which drugs are used and how they are given. Side effects such as rash, fever, chills, or diarrhoea can happen in many people who have cancer and during chemotherapy treatment. Most of these side effects go away when treatment is over, but you should always report any unusual symptoms right away to your nurse or doctor.

Does chemotherapy make you more tired?

You may be extra tired after this kind of treatment, so ask for help as you need it.

What are the side effects?

Side effects depend on the type of chemotherapy and how it is given. However, the most common side effects are fatigue, nausea, vomiting, and diarrhoea.

Who will treat me when I have chemo?

Your nurse will be responsible for giving the chemo treatment. Oncology social workers work with patients, families and doctors to support coping with cancer treatment side effects like pain and depression. Your physician or team may also prescribe medications that can help with side effects or other symptoms you might have during your cancer care.

Chemotherapy Treatment And Your Personality

The question seems to come up more and more as cancers are being diagnosed at earlier ages (or, in some cases, in older adults).

For instance, a recent study by Aarhus University Hospital in Denmark found that cancer survivors who had chemotherapy and radiation as children were five times more likely to be diagnosed with a personality disorder.

But what does the science say? First, it's essential to understand what chemotherapy does and doesn't do.

Chemotherapy is designed to attack fast-growing cells in your body—chiefly cancer cells. But chemotherapy drugs accidentally kill other rapidly dividing cells, including hair follicles and the intestinal tract lining.

So, the side effects are generally related to these types of damage—hair loss or changes in bowel function. But they can also include cognitive changes.

As I mentioned, we know that cancer survivors who had chemotherapy as children have a higher incidence of personality disorders. Some of the changes are associated with cognitive problems, such as brain fog and forgetfulness.

But once we got a look at the personality disorders among these cancer survivors, we noticed something else, and it was an interesting pattern. The more chemotherapy they received, the more likely they were to have a particular personality disorder called "borderline."

The borderline personality disorder doesn't give a damn; it's highly impulsive and shifts from one extreme to another. For instance, when a borderline person is angry, they will yell and scream. If you give them a small word of criticism, they might accuse you of disloyalty.

Some researchers think that the defining characteristic of borderline personality disorder is splitting behaviour—where people see themselves and others in "black or white" terms. One minute they're your best friend and then your worst enemy.

You may have experienced this phenomenon before. Perhaps you've known people who are extremely sensitive about small matters—very emotional. But even though they might often be your close friends, they will explode if you criticize the slightest thing or if you don't ascribe the same level of importance to your comments or opinions. You are either totally loved or wholly hated, and that is it.

And among people with borderline personality disorder, anger and irritability are quite common. They are quick to feel insulted and then to react with hostility—sometimes in a disproportionate manner.

And that's the pattern we saw in the cancer survivors who had a diagnosis of borderline personality disorder. They reported much higher irritability, frustration and anger than those who didn't have this diagnosis. They also had twice as much trouble controlling their anger as others did.

They also reported more problems with sadness and anxiety, but this was only true if they hadn't received chemotherapy to the head.

We confirmed that some of the cognitive symptoms associated with borderline personality disorder such as brain fog might be connected to chemotherapy.

But there are probably other factors involved, too, because they also reported more physical problems. For instance, they experienced more frequent heart palpitations and chest pain. And they had a three times greater risk for developing arthritis.

And these problems are usually worse in the long run. One of our team members has been studying cancer survivors for many years—most of the men—and he found that, compared to healthy people, those who had received chemotherapy during childhood were more than twice as likely to develop heart disease later in life.

But if you're not very familiar with the current medical literature, you might be wondering how we could connect cancer to borderline personality disorder. And the answer is that it is a genetic risk factor—so there may be a shared susceptibility. And also, chemotherapy treatments in childhood seem to be related to lower levels of brain development. So that might also be involved in the link.

In addition, the way we see things now is that while borderline personality disorder can cause many difficulties in life, they are not inherent to the condition. Instead, they are probably more directly connected with childhood trauma and abuse than to anything else.

For example, a study of almost 1,400 patients found that 96% reported emotional abuse before the age of 18—and 89% physical abuse. And an extensive study found that people with BPD were six times more likely to have suffered childhood sexual abuse or neglect than healthy people. And I believe this abuse is also connected to the high rates of suicide in BPD and their higher-than-average risk for cancer.

So whenever you have an unpleasant experience in life, especially in childhood. You can call this a "flashback" when you imagine the past. And a flashback is an extreme version of what we call " daydreaming."

These are highly emotional, vivid images and memories that you're having right now that are connected to something in your past. They're very intense, and they come up unexpectedly. But if you're familiar with your mind and body, they also happen often enough for you to know what they feel like.

Chemo Brain

What is a chemo brain?

Also is known as cognitive dysfunction, it is a condition where some patients undergoing chemotherapy develop mild problems with concentration, memory, and word-finding.

You may also have difficulty focusing your attention on one task at a time and controlling your impulses. Additionally, some people may experience generalized anxiety (feeling anxious all the time), irritability, fatigue or insomnia (having trouble sleeping).

The severity of these symptoms can vary from mild to severe.

Chemotherapy brain symptoms usually last a few months following your chemotherapy treatment is completed. There is no known treatment for chemo brain.

Most people who develop a chemo brain also have some other problems with their thinking, memory, or concentration.

What are the symptoms of chemotherapy brain?

The symptoms of chemotherapy brain may include:

cognitive fatigue - where you feel tired and have difficulties with concentration, focus and memory.

Inability to concentrate – You may find it hard to stay alert over some time.

Mood changes – You may feel irritable, depressed or anxious (especially towards the end of treatment or after stopping treatment).

The more you have chemotherapy brain, the longer the symptoms last.

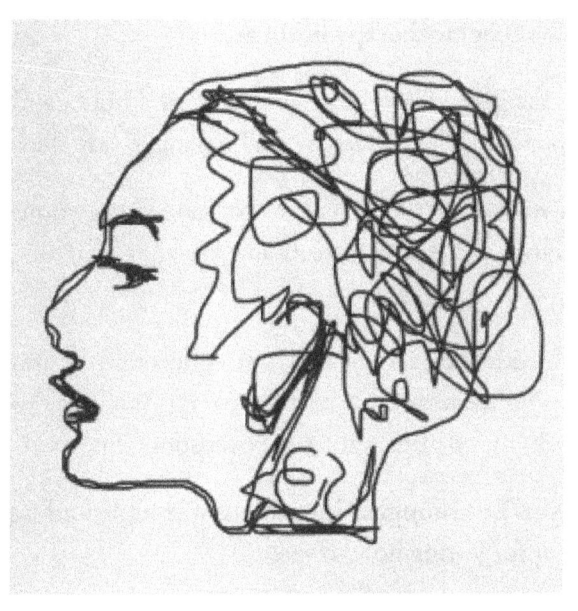

The main types of chemotherapy brain are:

1. **Cognitive fatigue**: from the pressure to think and concentrate too much, where it can be challenging to stay alert.

2. **Changes in mood**: feeling irritable, depressed or anxious (especially towards the end of treatment or after stopping treatment).

3. **Difficulty thinking clearly** – a lack of concentration and poor memory/concentration problems & ability to concentrate/focus on one thing at a time over some time.

4. **The inability to put thoughts into words** – trouble finding the right word or forgetting how to spell.

5. **Confusion** - forgetfulness, disorientation and feeling fuzzy-headed, so your brain feels dull and foggy.

Who is at risk?

Most people who are undergoing chemotherapy for cancer develop some symptoms of chemo brain. However, certain people are more at risk:

The older you get, the more likely you are to develop a chemo brain (older age makes you more vulnerable).

People with low overall health may be more likely to have problems with their thinking, memory or concentration.

Also, women do not have a higher risk of having problems with thinking, memory or concentration.

What is chemo brain treatment?

There is no known cure for chemo brain, and most people can tolerate the symptoms with some medication.

Your oncologist or nurse can help you work out how long you will need to take each type of medication and decide on a plan to deal with these symptoms at home. Depending on your particular needs, you may need advice from a specialist doctor about coping with the side effects.

Chemotherapy Equipment Used

- An oncologist administers this treatment into the vein via a catheter inserted in the patient's vein. It goes directly to the cancer cells, killing them.

- Chemotherapy can be administered at a hospital or clinic, or home. The latter occurs when patients are given instructions as to how and when to self-administer treatment. If administering chemotherapy at home, follow all of the oncologist's instructions carefully.

If you have any questions about administering treatments at home, call your medical provider.

What are the side effects of chemotherapy?

- Side effects depend on the type and dose of chemotherapy given and each patient's response to the treatment. They may include but are not limited to nausea and vomiting, hair loss, diarrhoea, mouth sores and fatigue. These side effects usually occur during or shortly after treatment and can be managed with medications.

- Side effects from chemotherapy are usually temporary and go away once treatment is completed. However, they may become less tolerable as time goes by. If you experience any severe side effects that you cannot manage using medication or relaxation techniques (such as deep breathing), notify your doctor immediately.

- Chemotherapy is a standard treatment method for some types of cancer. While some side effects of chemotherapy are inevitable, they can usually be effectively managed – even eliminated – using medication or relaxation techniques such as deep breathing.

What are the side effects caused by chemotherapy?

- Chemotherapy can affect the entire body, but its effects can be managed by reducing or eliminating side effects via medication or relaxation techniques like deep breathing.

- Some of the most common side effects include nausea and vomiting, hair loss, mouth sores and fatigue. Patients may feel nauseous because of chemotherapy going through their vein to their heart and lungs. They may also vomit due to a poor reaction to certain medications. The process of vomiting will be uncomfortable, so they must take medication to minimize the problem. In addition, hair loss can occur because this treatment affects all cells, including those in the roots of human hair shafts, which led to thinning of hair that falls out when combing or brushing.

Stage 1 Cancer And Chemotherapy

Yes. Even Stage 1 cancers are often treated with a chemotherapy drug called Adriamycin (chemical name: Doxorubicin), along with radiation therapy.

What are the goals of chemotherapy?

Chemotherapy uses anti-cancer drugs to stop or slow the growth of cancer cells and lessen symptoms such as pain or tiredness from cancer that has spread to other areas of your body.

The Success Rate Of Chemotherapy

The success rate of chemotherapy varies according to the type of cancer being treated. However, the potential for success with a carefully selected treatment program is fairly high.

What You Should Not Do During Chemotherapy

Do not drive. Not even go to work. Your oncologist or nurse will tell you what days and hours to take off from work or school. Your oncologist or nurse will also tell you how long to be out of work, but you should not stop working entirely until your oncologist tells you it is OK. But will probably want to know how she is doing with chemotherapy as well.

For example, if your test results show that your blood counts are low, you may be admitted to the hospital for a few days for treatment with medications or blood transfusions. Your oncologist will explain what this means. You may also be given drugs to strengthen your immune system and help keep infections from developing. It is normal for you to feel tired and weak after chemotherapy, so make sure you rest as much as possible when you are in the hospital.

What should you do during chemotherapy?

It is not suitable to receive chemotherapy treatments during an infection. This may weaken your immune system. However, your doctor will tell you what kind of infection you are infected with and when it is OK to have chemotherapy treatments.

It is not recommended that you receive chemotherapy during your pregnancy. However, you may receive chemotherapy during this time if your health would be in danger or if cancer could spread to other organs of your body.

You should let your doctor know if you are pregnant and do not think about getting pregnant for at least a year after you stop receiving chemotherapy treatment if you have breast cancer.

Boosting Your Immune System During Chemotherapy

No question about it: Chemotherapy is tough on your immune system. At the same time, your immune system plays an essential role in fighting cancer, so keeping it as healthy as possible is extremely important and not just during chemotherapy treatment. At any given time, your body is continuously exposed to bacteria and viruses that can be harmful to you.

Your immune system's job is to fight off these invaders before they have a chance to cause problems for you. That's why it's so important to take steps to help your immune system work at its best—not just during chemotherapy but every day.

To help protect your immune system:

Get vaccinated. The flu vaccine is a great example. It's not just for people who are currently sick with the flu. It can also help prevent you from developing flu symptoms in the first place by building up your body's natural defences.

The flu vaccine is a great example. It's not just for people who are currently sick with the flu. It can also help prevent you from developing flu symptoms in the first place by building up your body's natural defences. Eat a healthy diet. Fruits and vegetables are high in vitamins and minerals like vitamin C, which can help boost your immune system.

Fruits and vegetables are high in vitamins and minerals like vitamin C, which can help boost your immune system. Get enough sleep. Sleep helps keep your immune system working well so it can fight off any infection you might come into contact with the next day.

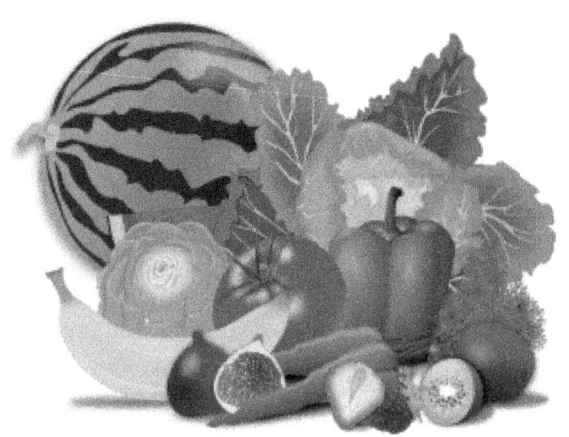

Rest

Sleep helps keep your immune system working well so it can fight off any infection you might come into contact with the next day. Be physically active. Exercise is another excellent way to boost your immune system. It can help keep your body healthy and strong.

Exercise is another excellent way to boost your immune system. It can help keep your body healthy and strong. Keep stress under control. Stress can suppress the immune system, making you more likely to get sick. Cut down on sources of stress in your life whenever possible to keep from getting overwhelmed by them.

Staying well during chemotherapy is extremely important for helping you recover as quickly as possible. The best thing you can do for yourself during treatment is to practice good self-care—which includes staying as relaxed and stress-free as you can, eating a healthy diet, getting enough rest, and staying physically active for 30 minutes a day or more each week. It's also a good idea to see a doctor about other things that can help you recover faster, such as using exercise or meditation to reduce stress.

Cancer and chemo treatment are viciously trying on the body, which can make it difficult for your diet to keep up.

Your appetite may be off; you might struggle with nausea, or you may not have enough strength in your stomach to eat anything solid. But food is even more important than usual when fighting cancer, so don't just depend on what feels good at any given moment and hope it will do the trick.

Most cancer treatments are provided as a drug, such as chemotherapy, so a healthy diet is also necessary for the body to absorb those drugs.

Before you change your diet, consult with your doctor to find out what foods are good for you and which ones aren't. Some foods that may be alright include poultry, fish and eggs; fruit and vegetables; whole grains; beans; nuts and seeds; legumes (like lentils); low-fat dairy products; olive oil. Avoid high-fat foods, and limit your alcohol intake.

What to drink?

Water is the best choice to help keep your body hydrated and flush out the drugs that are being given. Rather than put fruit juice in your water or add anything else to it (including cucumber or other fruit skin), try diluting it with an equal amount of water. This will ensure you're getting the right liquid that has good vitamins and minerals.

To help your body absorb the drugs, it's a good idea to drink a lot of water and eat little bits of food throughout the day, rather than all at once. A low-fat protein source such as yoghurt or steak is also fine.

If you are receiving chemo, you will want to remove oil from your food for a few days while on drugs to prevent nausea; you can also remove salt, garlic and citrus fruits for the same reason. Increase fluids into your system without adding extra sugars you don't need.

Avoid the following during chemo:

caffeine, alcohol and red meat. Caffeine makes it harder for patients to handle the effects of the drugs, and red meat is linked to an increased risk of heart disease. Alcohol can cause nausea by interfering with sleep and causing dehydration, so you might need to avoid it for a couple of days. If you do drink alcohol, stick with beer and wine don't mix it with cocktails or mixed drinks.

Always check with your oncology doctor and nutritionist.

Food For Chemotherapy And Radiation Therapy Cancer Treatment In General

The food you eat has a direct effect on the outcome of your chemotherapy and radiation therapy treatment. Therefore, proper nutrition is essential during cancer treatment and what you can do to get adequate nutrition.

Cancer patients who undergo chemotherapy and radiation therapy need to follow a special diet plan. But this doesn't mean you need to make any significant changes to your current eating habits. It just means that you should make some minor adjustments to what you consume.

For example, the foods that are good for you in a normal daily diet should continue to be good in your diet during cancer treatment. The goal is to have your nutritional intake meet the recommended dietary allowance (RDA) for healthy people. RDA is a standard of ideal nourishment that can help prevent deficiency diseases and improve peak physical performance.

The following are the dietary guidelines for cancer patients undergoing chemotherapy and radiation therapy:

Good Diets During Chemotherapy And Radiation Therapy Cancer Treatment

Eat a lot of fruits and vegetables

Choose fruits over juices (especially apricot and prune juices)

Eat whole fruit instead of drinking fruit juice. Fruit juices contain more sugar than whole fruits do, so use them in moderation. You can get your daily requirement of vitamins and minerals by eating two to three servings of fruits or vegetables each day.

Eat many nutritious carbohydrates, such as whole-grain kinds of pasta, yams, brown rice, and potatoes.

Eat healthy fats. Eating healthy fats does not make you gain weight as long as you eat the right kinds of fats and in the right amounts. Good choices include fish oils, nuts and seeds, olive oil, and olives.

Use herbs and spices to enhance the taste of your diet rather than to mask its flavour. Herbs and spices are loaded with powerful antioxidants, which help to protect your body from free radical damage.

Grill or broil food rather than frying it in oil. Studies have shown that cooking food with a dry heat source is healthier than cooking with a wet heat source because the drier heat helps maintain more nutrients in the food.

Eat lean meats, low-fat dairy products, and smaller portions of meat. In addition, you can add healthy fats back into your diet by eating fish and nuts.

Be careful of the condiments you choose. Spicy brown mustard, garlic salt, and ketchup contain high amounts of sodium. You are better off choosing salsa and fresh fruit to flavour your meat.

Choose lemons or limes over salt when you need to add some flavour to a dish.

Is Chemotherapy Working

———

A complete response means that all signs of cancer have disappeared, and the tumour has shrunk. So you may return to your everyday activities.

A partial response means that your tumour has shrunk by at least 30%. You will continue with the chemotherapy treatment that caused the reaction.

An objective response means that your tumour has shrunk by at least 30%. The doctor cannot feel or see any tumour tissue. A CT scan, PET scan or physical exam may reveal any remaining cancer cells.

You will continue with the chemotherapy treatment that produced the response.

The Pros And Cons Of Chemotherapy Treatment

No matter what kind of chemotherapy you are receiving, the treatment will cause a lot of symptoms. Most of these symptoms are related to your immune system. That's because chemotherapy will try to wipe out any cancer cells in your body and make them inactive.

Chemotherapy may also damage healthy cells throughout your body. This is because it tries to destroy all the cancer cells in your body. These side effects are called complications. Minor complications can pass as your immune system tries to recover from the chemo drugs. However, severe complications may cause you to need more treatment.

As a patient, what can you do to help with the symptoms and complications?

First, try not to be in pain or discomfort. Second, you'll want to stay strong for your body and your immune system, so take small breaks whenever you can.

Finally, try to stay relaxed and comfortable. It would help if you were healthy for your body to fight off cancer cells and complications.

Here is a list of things you can do, if possible:

You'll want to stay hydrated during treatment, especially when you're receiving chemotherapy drugs. These drugs will dehydrate your body pretty quickly. Staying hydrated will help you feel better, especially when you suffer from side effects like nausea (feeling sick). Drink water whenever you can or use oral rehydration solutions (ORS).

ORS can be found at pharmacies and will help hydrate your body quickly, especially if you start feeling nauseous or are suffering from diarrhoea.

If you have trouble urinating, you may need to take a "urinal". This is a bedside tool that will help you urinate more efficiently. You may also experience pain in your bladder area, which makes it hard to urinate without the help of a "urinal".

In addition to water, stay hydrated with plenty of fruit juices and flavoured water to rehydrate your body during chemotherapy. Fruit juices are also high in vitamins and minerals that can help boost your immune system.

If you're receiving chemo treatment combined with radiation, you will also need to drink plenty of water.

The radiation will dehydrate your body that much more. Your oncologist or nurse will let you know how much water to drink each day to stay healthy and hydrated during treatment.

Your mouth may also become dry and painful as a result of chemotherapy. You may need to gargle with warm salt water (1 tsp salt in 1 cup warm water) to moisten your mouth and throat area. Sipping on this mixture throughout the day can help soothe your throat, so it doesn't become painful when you swallow.

You may experience changes in the way your skin feels. For example, you may have red spots on your skin, and your skin could become very dry. Try moisturizing with vegetable oils, such as jojoba oil, once or twice a day.

Chemotherapy And Long-Term Damage

The short-term side effects from chemotherapy usually go away after treatment is over. Some late side effects are possible, but they are rare. For example, some people have fertility problems after chemotherapy, or their hair never grows back.

Foods That Help Shrink Tumours

Vegetables:

A variety of healthy vegetables can be added to your diet. These include artichokes, asparagus, broccoli, cabbage, cauliflower, and kale. Besides being a great source of protein and fibre, these vegetables also contain antioxidants that help fight cancerous cells and tumours.

Fruits:

Berries contain large amounts of phytochemicals like ellagic acid, which slows tumour growth. Other fruits that are important in this process are apples and orange.

Note: *Green tea contains natural cancer-fighting substances.*

What foods interfere with chemotherapy?

Foods that interfere with cancer treatment because can cause an immune response that destroys the cancer cells.

These include dairy products and wheat products. When drinking milk, it is advisable to do so while fasting to avoid a sickness of some sort. Also, try not to drink milk unless you have a cold or sore throat; this will help prevent the sickness from developing into something more serious. Also, when eating bread and pasta, it is best to avoid wheat and sometimes rice as well but first, always check with your chemo nutritionist and oncologist.

What is the alternative to chemotherapy treatment?

The National Cancer Institute (NCI) has a list of available alternative options to the standard course of chemotherapy. This list also includes more than 40 research studies that show the effectiveness of these alternative treatment options.

Some alternatives to chemotherapy include:

There is not a single cure for cancer, but many complementary and alternative therapies are being studied to determine their usefulness as a cancer treatment. In some cases, these treatments have been studied for years. One example is the use of vitamins B3 and B6.

Many medications have been used to treat various cancers, but their effectiveness varies from one disease to another. For example, it is not known whether the blood pressure medication Captopril will treat cancer of the prostate or if estrogen will work for breast cancer. Because of this, doctors often combine several different medicines to get the best results possible for each patient's cancer.

After surgery, some treatments can help prevent the spread of cancer cells and increase the chances of a cure. For example:

What is immunotherapy?

Immunotherapy is a way to stimulate a person's immune system to fight off disease. These drugs are being used in the treatment of many kinds of cancer. Some examples are:

Many people choose "alternative treatments" instead of standard cancer treatment because they think they are more natural than drugs and other therapies that the medical community usually recommends. The word "natural" is used to describe both foods and alternative therapies. Some people use alternative medicine to cure their disease, while others use it to treat symptoms.

However, many natural substances are harmful. And, all-natural therapies have not been researched as well as some conventional treatments.

If you choose an alternative treatment instead of standard cancer treatment, be sure that the therapy has been proven effective or that research is being done on the treatment.

Researching Complementary and Alternative therapies

Many organizations provide information on cancer and complementary and alternative cancer treatments. These organizations include the National Cancer Institute (NCI), the American Cancer Society (ACS), the American College of Surgeons, and the National Institutes of Health. When planning what treatments to use, you should research all kinds of treatment options.

There are many of these organizations that can help you research complementary and alternative treatments. For example, the Cancer Resource Center at Columbia University teaches people how to research themselves and find resources. Also, the National Cancer Institute provides several educational tools through its website, including an online publication called Guide to Complementary and Alternative Treatments.

The "*Cancer Treatment Advisor*" section of the National Cancer Institute website includes detailed information about complementary and alternative treatments in cancer care.

"*Cancer treatment is not a one-drug fix. The more choices, the better.*" "The challenge we face with cancer is that people are surprised when they learn that the standard of care for many types of cancers is nothing more than it has always been. For some adult cancers, no alternative medicine therapy has ever shown to be safe and effective."

In addition, the authors of a Cochrane review found "No high-quality evidence base exists to support the use of any complementary and alternative therapy in adults with cancer. There is no evidence to support the use of acupuncture, aromatherapy, massage therapy and other non-cultural and non-drug interventions for any cancer type."

Various complementary treatments are not well supported by research, and there is little clinical evidence that any effective complementary treatment has ever been shown to be safe and effective. This lack of adequate evidence was affirmed in a Cochrane review published in May 2007 that reviewed 12 randomized controlled trials on therapies with potentially plausible mechanisms of action. The review found that only hypericum (St John's wort) was associated with a statistically significant antidepressant effect, albeit a modest one compared to the standard drug treatment.

The use of antineoplastons is an unapproved cancer therapy sold by the Burzynski Research Institute, Texas, USA. The FDA does not approve the therapy. However, the company has run an international clinical trials network since 1977. Some of these trials have been peer-reviewed and published in journals such as Cancer Research.

The use of antineoplastons is an unapproved cancer therapy sold by the Burzynski Research Institute, Texas, USA. The FDA does not approve the therapy. However, the company has run an international clinical trials network since 1977. Some of these trials have been peer-reviewed and published in journals such as Cancer Research.

Antineoplastons are a biological response modifier used mainly in the treatment of chronic myeloid leukaemia (CML). In CML treatment, they are combined with conventional chemotherapy and interferon-alpha therapy. Stanislaw Burzynski originally developed them in the 1970s as part of a cancer gene therapy research program.

In 1981, Burzynski published the results of an in vivo study that showed that antineoplastons could slow down the progression of a patient's disease. In 1984, Burzynski was awarded a research grant to continue his work on anti-tumour activity. As a result, he began to use antineoplastons (produced in large batches by extraction from the urine of patients) as an adjunct to chemotherapy. His laboratory has published more than 250 peer-reviewed scientific papers on the topic. In addition, the results of these trials have been widely reproduced and discussed in other medical journals, including the New England Journal of Medicine (NEJM) and Lancet (a British Medical Journal).

Antineoplastons are synthesized from human urine. The formula for antineoplaston A10, as described in the United States Patent and Trademark Office, is:

The patent quotes the following:

However, the patent does not state how A-10 forms or is formed in urine.

Burzynski's therapy consists of a long list of ingredients that other researchers have found to be potentially toxic or ineffective. For example, there have been no peer-reviewed papers supporting the effectiveness of glucarolactone or methylglyoxal (also known as M.G.). Also, some of the other ingredients are potentially toxic, ineffective or used for the wrong disease or situation. These include aloe vera (not effective), bilberry extract (used in eye health and wound healing; not supported by research in improving the immune system). Chinese herbs and mushrooms such as Cordyceps sinensis, Ganoderma lucidum and Lingzhi (unsupported by research for cancer treatment; can cause fungal infection; may also be used to treat asthma rather than cancer). Ginkgo Biloba (possibly effective for eye health; ineffective for immune function, possibly harmful if combined with steroids), soy protein and Spirulina platensis.

A 2012 review by the Cochrane Collaboration concluded, "Provisional evidence suggests that using antineoplaston therapy may be associated with improving some measures of well-being. However, the effects on quality of life and disease-free survival are too small to be meaningful."

Burzynski's website states that: "The more choices, the better." It also encourages its patients to ask for a complete treatment plan. A patient benefits from this approach by getting access to a wide range of complementary and alternative cancer treatments. In this way, combining complementary and alternative therapies with conventional cancer treatment increases patient options while reducing the financial burden.

Dr Burzynski treats cancer with antineoplastons, a substance produced in the human body, which has been successfully used as a cancer treatment since the 1970s. The antineoplastons are molecular fragments of proteins found in normal body functions (i.e. neurotransmitters, peptides and amino acids).

Currently, antineoplaston therapy can be prescribed for almost every type of cancer. The list of malignancies treated by Dr Burzynski's therapy includes:

For many of these cancers, alternative medicine has been shown to be effective and complementary treatment regimens have been shown to provide added benefit.

While the FDA has approved antineoplastons as a cancer treatment since 1981, the only U.S. study to date has been completed by Dr Burzynski and his research team at Baylor College of Medicine in 1990.

The study was published in the New England Journal of Medicine in 1991 and showed that antineoplastons were effective at treating cancer when used with other standard therapies. In addition, Dr Burzynski's FDA-approved Phase II trial has been replicated and published.

The results also showed a significant decrease in blood transfusions and improvement of quality of life. In addition, the study demonstrated that antineoplastons could be combined with other standard therapies, including radiation therapy, chemotherapy or interferon-alpha.

Dr Burzynski has also completed eight Phase III/IV trials, all of which have been peer-reviewed and published in journals such as Cancer Research, the New England Journal of Medicine and the Lancet.

The results showed that antineoplastons could be combined with other standard therapies, including radiation therapy, chemotherapy and immunotherapy. This combination treatment has been shown to improve quality of life and increase the chance of survival time. Dr Burzynski has completed eight Phase III/IV trials since the late 1980s, all peer-reviewed and published in journals such as Cancer Research, the New England Journal of Medicine and the Lancet.

In 1995, Dr Burzynski's antineoplaston therapy was shown to be effective at treating Glioblastoma Multiforme (GBM), the most aggressive form of brain tumour.

According to Dr Burzynski, the results of his study show that antineoplaston therapy can be used as a complementary treatment for cancer. The study also showed a significant decrease in the need for blood transfusions and improvement of quality of life.

Combining Supplementing Treatment With Alternative Therapies

The American Cancer Society reports that over a million Americans, a year, receive chemotherapy for cancer treatment. Chemotherapy is designed to kill cancer cells and stop them from growing so the body can get rid of them. Unfortunately, chemo can also hurt healthy cells along with the cancerous ones that are targeted. This is what causes the side effects of nausea, vomiting, and hair loss. Alternative therapies may help relieve some of these side effects, so you have a more tolerable experience during chemotherapy treatment.

Alternatives to chemotherapy can include:

· Herbal therapy- supplements that are made of plants that have a calming effect on the nervous system.

· acupuncture is a natural technique that involves inserting thin needles into specific body areas for pain relief.

Acupuncture has been proven to effectively lower anxiety and lowers the pain level in patients who undergo chemotherapy.

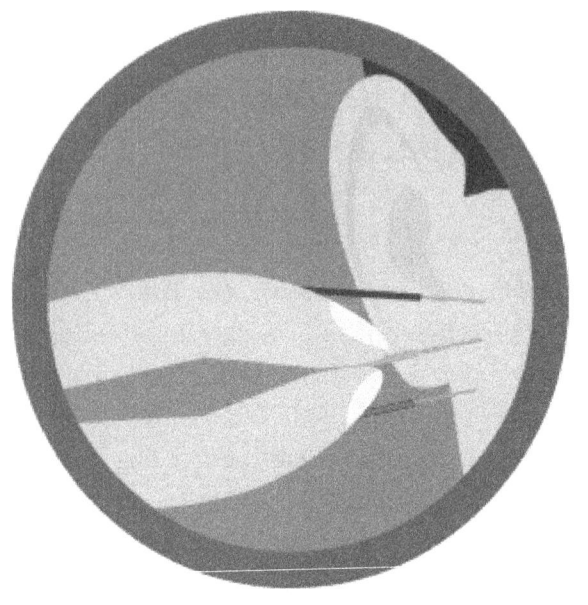

- Massage therapy- which is a natural method for pain relief and relaxation.

- yoga- a form of exercise that promotes relaxation and meditation. It also promotes cancer healing and general well-being.

Can you have a massage after cancer treatment?

A qualified massage therapist can provide you with gentle, therapeutic massage during and after cancer treatment. See more about massage therapy after cancer treatment.

Can you practice yoga?

Yes, a qualified yoga teacher can teach you a wide variety of safe exercises to accompany your chemotherapy as a complementary cancer treatment alternative. Read more about yoga therapy during chemotherapy treatment.

What is the difference between Western medicine and alternative medicine? Western medicine is based upon scientific knowledge and is very effective at diagnosing and treating medical conditions. Western medicine includes allopathic, osteopathic, chiropractic and other medical disciplines. Alternative medicine is any practice that is a non-invasive treatment option to treat cancer. Alternative treatments include herbal remedies, homoeopathic remedies, and other non-conventional therapies.

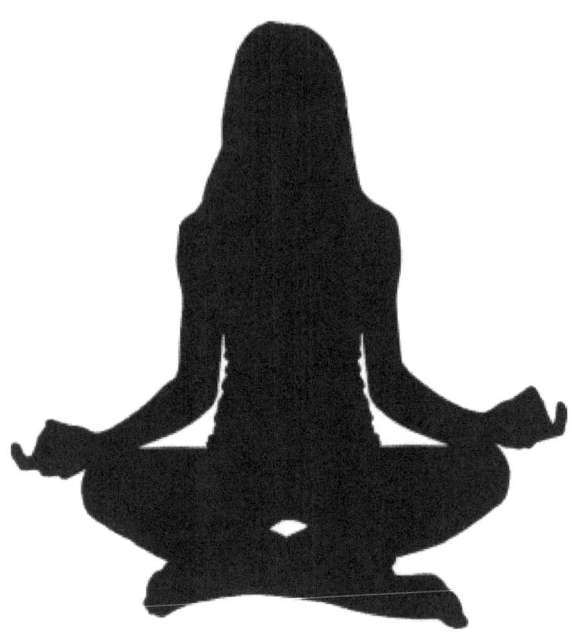

Due to the side effects of chemotherapy, many people are uncomfortable with continuing their treatment. In truth, alternative therapies can help supplement your chemotherapy treatment plan so you can get the most out of your chemotherapy sessions.

You may recall in the first section. Did I mention ChemoActive?

What is ChemoActive?

ChemoActive is the first-ever nutritional supplement clinically proven to reduce side effects and increase patient comfort during cancer treatment. This proprietary formula has a unique combination of nutrients, enzymes and botanicals, which work together to ensure that patients experience less pain, lower incidence of nausea, vomiting and fatigue while receiving their chemotherapy and radiation treatments.

The Food & Drug Administration (FDA) recognizes ChemoActive as a dietary supplement. This means that the product is classified as a food in the United States and can be sold to consumers without prior approval from the FDA.

ChemoActive is not a drug and has not been tested or approved by the FDA to prevent or treat any illness, disease, injury, or other condition.

What are the ingredients of ChemoActive?

ChemoActive contains a proprietary blend of active plant-based minerals, phytonutrients, enzymes and botanicals.

This proprietary blend has been specifically designed to support the immune system while inhibiting the side effects of chemotherapy and radiation therapy.

What are Phytonutrients?

Phytonutrients are naturally occurring compounds that are essential to the health and vitality of all living things. They act as catalysts to "turn on" the body's self-healing systems.

What are the benefits of Phytonutrients?

When taken in combination with enzymes and supporting minerals, phytonutrients can provide an instant defence against the damaging side effects of chemotherapy. They have also been clinically proven to significantly increase energy levels and reduce fatigue during chemotherapy treatment.

Alternative Complementary Cancer Treatments

The National Cancer Institute provides excellent information and a list of organizations for finding alternative cancer treatment options. An ideal place to start your search for an alternative cancer treatment program is at the NCI's website or directly at the National Center for Alternative and Integrative Health.

What is holistic medical treatment?

Holistic medical treatment is a well-integrated approach to diagnosing, treating, and rehabilitating physical disorders by combining conventional and complementary medicine.

What is complementary medicine?

Complementary medicine refers to any therapy that supplements what is already known about healing the body through conventional treatment.

Can you take acupuncture during chemotherapy treatment?

Although much research has been done on acupuncture for cancer treatment, there is no proof that this complementary cancer treatment is more effective than Western medicine alone.

Can alternative cancer treatments help with the side effects of conventional chemo?

In a limited number of cases, alternative cancer treatments can help to reduce or eliminate the side effects of chemotherapy, such as nausea and hair loss.

Can you have massage therapy during chemotherapy treatment?

A qualified massage therapist can provide you with gentle, therapeutic massage during and after cancer treatment.

Can you practice yoga during chemotherapy treatment?

Yes, a qualified yoga teacher can teach you a wide variety of safe exercises to accompany your chemotherapy as a complementary cancer treatment alternative.

Many conditions may have symptoms similar to those of cancer. This is especially true if the symptoms are new and have not been ongoing for some time. Other names used for these conditions are "false positives" or "noncancerous". This means that you may be put on chemo or radiation for a condition that is not cancer. There are several reasons why a physician may do so. The most common are:

A doctor will only tell you that you have cancer if confirmed by a physical exam, biopsy or other tests.

Other tests used in the diagnosis of cancer include:

The distinction between malignant, benign and non-malignant tissue can be difficult to make during the early stages of diagnosis. Therefore, these three categories are used in the diagnosis of cancer.

Malignancy describes a tumour that can invade surrounding tissues and spread to other areas of the body. The doctor will use several tests to determine if your tumour is malignant or benign.

Non-malignant tumours generally do not spread beyond the organ where they originated. Non-malignant tumours may require treatment, but not usually chemotherapy or radiation therapy, which are used to treat malignancies and cancer.

Malignant tumours are tested with one or more of the following tests:

Aggressive tumours have invaded surrounding tissue and can spread to other areas of the body. Aggressive tumours may also have a strong likelihood of metastasizing, which is when they spread (metastasize) to other areas of the body where they can cause harm. Aggressive tumours may require treatment, particularly chemo or radiation therapy.

Some examples of aggressive tumours:

Which treatment you choose will depend on various factors, including your age, location and type of cancer, general health, and family medical history. Treatment may involve surgery to remove some or all of the cancer, radiation therapy to control the growth of cancer cells or chemotherapy to control the growth of cancer cells.

+ (positive) = growth; - (negative) = no growth.

Lymphomas, haematological cancers and solid tumours, are immunogenic diseases, i.e. they make the body's immune system attack the cancerous cells as if they were an infection.

Effective treatment can be achieved by anti-inflammatory drugs and by immunoablation (removal of part or all of the immune system).

Immunoablation involves the destruction of the immune system through various methods, which are generally considered unethical. These methods include chemotherapy in which cancerous cells are destroyed through exposure to chemotherapeutic agents, radiation therapy, and cryotherapy (freezing). The very purpose of this modality is to essentially cut off a part of your body's natural defences against cancerous cells.

These treatments have shortcomings since they do not address the cause of cancerous cells remaining in the body. They also involve significant collateral damage to the whole body. In all cases, immunoablation shakes the immune system of a human being into submission; it is ridden with potentially fatal side effects. Furthermore, it does not address the cause of cancer but suppresses symptoms.

However, immunoablation may be the only choice of treatment for certain forms of cancer. This may be due to a particular form of cancer's resistance to the conventional therapies or because a patient's health is so poor that chemotherapy and radiation would be too destructive or toxic.

With immunoablation, the primary objective is to eliminate all cancerous cells in an otherwise healthy body. While this is not achievable, the treatment can "cure" 90% or more patients. The remaining 10% or so will have to return to a cycle of chemotherapy and be immunoablated again.

Immunoablation is not a new idea; it was developed in the 1950s and 1960s. It was then superseded by chemotherapy and radiation therapy because it made people too sick to survive. More modern techniques have improved outcome significantly, the level of side effects has been reduced, and there is now a much wider choice of treatments available. However, the cost of this treatment is very high, and until the medical expenses of many modern diseases are reduced, its use will remain limited.

Radiation used in cancer therapy has three basic types: X-rays, gamma rays and charged particle beams. The most common form of radiation therapy used to treat cancer is X-ray radiation. X-rays are a form of electromagnetic radiation. Electromagnetic radiation consists of waves that oscillate at right angles to the direction of travel of the wave and at right angles to any magnetic field present. X-ray machines produce beams of X-ray electromagnetic radiation.

X-rays are used to treat cancer because they can penetrate some distance into human tissue, where they cause damage to the

DNA inside body cells. This form of damage may lead to cell death (apoptosis) or changes in gene function. These changes can lead to cell death, and new cells that haven't been affected by X-rays may grow in their place. These new cells do not have the same DNA and often have different expression of genes. With time, they will start to die due to the lack of genetic information (mutations).

The radiation dose required for effective treatment is very high. The higher the dose, the greater the chance of side effects. Radiation can have significant side effects such as nausea, vomiting, fatigue and hair loss.

Radiation is usually given in a hospital or outpatient clinic several times per week over several weeks or months. The health care team will work with you to ensure that your treatment is as comfortable as possible.

Several types of radiation therapy are used to treat cancer: The principal side effect of cancer radiotherapy is forming a hard collar around the neck from fibrosis, and sometimes, blood clots. The most common types are:

Radiation can also cause infertility in females and sterility in males. Therefore, if it is necessary to have sperm or oocytes preserved before radiotherapy treatment, they should be preserved as soon as possible after diagnosis, before radiation therapy.

Cancer cells can mutate to be resistant to radiation treatment.

Surgery is an integral part of any complete cancer treatment plan. Surgeons offer different methods of cancer surgery or treatments that include:

Adjuvant therapy is another form of cancer treatment that is important because it can help control certain cancers. Adjuvant therapy may be used after a tumour is removed by surgery. Doctors prescribe adjuvant therapies to help lower the risk of recurrence and improve the chance for cure in some patients diagnosed with late-stage disease. Adjuvant therapies are given along with primary radiation treatments.

Chemotherapy is considered an adjuvant treatment in some cancers, although the term usually applies to cancer prevention. It is a treatment given after surgery or radiation therapy to kill any remaining cancer cells that did not respond to the other treatments. Chemotherapy is recommended for use with certain cancers, such as testicular germ cell tumours, ovarian germ cell tumours, Hodgkin lymphoma, and various leukaemias and sarcomas.

The National Cancer Institute recommends combination chemotherapy to treat people with advanced-stage breast cancer or stage III or stage IV colon cancer.

Chemotherapy may be used when cancer is found late, and doctors think that cancer has already spread through the body. Chemotherapy does not cure a disease. It is used to rid the body of any remaining cancer cells if no other treatment could.

The three types of chemotherapy are:

Chemotherapy may be used before surgery to shrink a cancerous tumour's size and make it easier to remove. In breast cancer, chemotherapy can also be used to reduce the risk that cancer will return after surgery or radiation therapy. This is because cancer cells are most likely to grow in regions where healthy cells have been damaged or destroyed (the body's natural immune response tends to eliminate normal cells in these areas). Chemotherapy may help destroy abnormal and potentially dangerous cells in these same areas.

Chemotherapy can also help reduce the size of cancer to allow for a better chance of surgery or radiation therapy to work. Chemotherapy may also be used before surgery or radiation therapy because it stops recurrence (cancer coming back) after surgery by killing off any remaining cancer cells which may have survived.

In older women, chemotherapy may be used before surgery. This is particularly important when there are no good options for the type and stage of cancer. In these cases, certain forms of chemotherapy may be used before surgery.

Chemotherapy is also called "*chemo*". The most common types of chemotherapy used to treat cancer are: alkylating agents, nitrogen mustards, and antimetabolites such as Cytoxan or Mitomycin C. Alkylating agents are the most commonly used chemotherapy in the United States for advanced-stage cancers. They cause damage to DNA by breaking apart chemical bonds (amino acids) in DNA. In addition, because they are cell-cycle nonspecific, they can often kill rapidly dividing cells such as cancer cells.

A new form of chemotherapy has been developed in recent years. This is called targeted therapy. It is more specific than standard chemotherapy because it targets only cancer cells and does not damage healthy cells. Many drugs fall into this category so that each medication can be used to treat different types of cancer. The drugs are called anti-cancer agents. These are all drugs that have been proven to be effective at killing cancer cells.

The use of specific types of targeted therapies has given cancer treatment new levels of precision and control and has improved the lives of many patients with advanced-stage cancers.

Targeted therapies have been found to reduce the death rate in those who have aggressive forms of cancer, especially when combined with other treatments such as surgery and radiation therapy or palliative care.

Many targeted therapies are now available, including:

Targeted therapies are more specific than other types of chemotherapy. They can be accommodating when there is little or no evidence of cancer cells in the blood, bone marrow or tissues of the body known as the sentinel node. The use of targeted therapy can also be helpful for lung cancer, prostate cancer, melanoma and brain cancers that do not show signs in the early stages.

Targeted therapy alone is not always a good option for treating advanced-stage cancer, especially when the cancer is spreading. This may be because targeted therapies are only effective on certain cancers and do not work on all cancers. Or it may be because the targeted therapy had no effect on cancer at all and may even make it worse in some patients. This is why other treatments such as surgery and radiation therapy are still essential.

Targeted therapy is not always a good option for treating advanced-stage cancer, especially when the cancer is spreading. This may be because targeted therapies are only effective on certain cancers and do not work on all cancers. Or it may be because the targeted therapy had no effect on cancer at all and may even make it worse in some patients. This is why other treatments such as surgery and radiation therapy are still necessary.

Targeted therapies are also called 'drugs that target cancer cells. These are all drugs that have been proven to effectively kill cancer cells or slow cancer growth.

Targeted therapies can be used alone or combined with other treatments, including surgery, radiation therapy or palliative care. They may be used as first-line treatment for some cancers or when other treatments are not working. For example, recently, this approach has been used for treating advanced-stage melanoma. It is also helpful for treating lung cancer, breast cancer, colorectal cancer and Hodgkin lymphoma.

Targeted therapies are very effective for many patients with advanced-stage cancers and, in some cases, can be used as first-line treatment. However, they are most often used as a second-line treatment after other chemotherapy or targeted therapy types have stopped working.

For example, targeted therapies may be helpful for those who have lung cancer, prostate cancer, melanoma and brain cancers that do not show signs in the early stages.

In some cases, certain types of targeted therapies can be used as first-line treatment for these cancers. These are known as 'curative therapies'. These treatments may be used if all other options have failed or when cancer has been found in the early stages, and there is a good chance that it can be cured.

Other examples of targeted therapies include:

In the United States, chemotherapy is used to treat almost 40 per cent of cancer patients. More than 50 per cent of cancer patients use radiation therapy. Surgery is used to treat only about seven per cent of cancers. Palliative care, or comfort care, is more likely used by advanced-stage cancer and those with lung cancer or pancreatic cancer. But it can be used in any patient with a terminal disease or diseases that cannot be cured using other treatments.

There are many new research areas into how to use chemotherapy, radiation therapy and targeted therapies to be more effective for treating cancer. The hope is that soon, these advances will help improve cancer treatment even further. This will allow more people to live longer, healthier lives with less risk of side effects.

The patient should begin chemotherapy by talking with their doctor about the pros and cons of this treatment. The patient should also speak with their doctor about the type of cancer and discuss the treatments available.

Is Chemotherapy Safe?

Chemotherapy is a very effective cancer treatment. It has a long history of use in treating many types of cancers. (See the Background section for more.) In general, doctors' treatment to kill cancer cells and destroy tumour (cancer) tissue by chemotherapy works better than any other type of treatment, including surgery or radiation therapy.

Chemotherapy is not as safe as it should be, and safety issues are significant to discuss with your doctor or nurse before your first chemotherapy treatment begins. You should ask about the safety of your specific type of chemotherapy. You will also want to discuss the risks and how to deal with them.

You should also ask your doctor about the possible side effects of chemotherapy before starting your first treatment. Also, you will want to know what signs and symptoms you need to watch for or report to your doctor or nurse so that you can get treatment right away if something bad happens.

In general, the greater the dose of chemotherapy you receive (the more chemo drugs), the greater the likelihood that your body will become very sick. Therefore, you should plan to have someone with you at all times while receiving chemotherapy so that if you become sick, they can take care of you.

The three most common types of chemotherapy are listed below. (These types of chemotherapy are used for "all" types of cancer.) There are many other types available for special situations.

Suppose you have a solid tumour (such as most forms of cancer). In that case, chemotherapy is the most likely treatment to cure your cancer, and it will be combined with surgery, radiation therapy, or a clinical trials drug. This type of treatment is sometimes called "combination treatment".

If you have a very rare type of cancer, you may be able to receive chemo treatment as a "standard of care" by an oncologist or other cancer specialist. This is called "monotherapy".

The doctors and nurses who take care of you during chemo treatment will tell you what to expect. However, you should read this information carefully and ask questions if you do not understand something.

Questions To Ask Before Chemotherapy Treatment

What questions do I need to ask the nurse or my doctor?

The doctor can offer two general chemotherapy treatments or chemotherapy treatments in combination. The specific chemotherapy use and choices for each treatment are based on the types of cancers, your health, and how your body responds to the drugs used.

Asking your physician questions can help ensure that you receive the best possible medical treatment. Your doctor will give you specific questions to ask about your illness, treatment plan, and test results.

What questions should I ask my doctor about my chemotherapy treatment?

When you find a doctor, who will be treating you with chemotherapy, there are some critical questions to ask:

- *What are the side effects of the specific drugs that your doctor has prescribed?*
- *When and how do the side effects usually occur?*
- *What is the best dose to give?*
- *Will I be hospitalized or treated in an outpatient facility?*

- *How long will treatment last? (This can vary from several weeks to several years.*
- *Will further treatmentsbe needed if the tumour is gone, but cancer has spread to another part of the body?*
- *What tests will be given before each treatment?*

When you ask your doctor questions about chemotherapy, **bring a list of questions** that you have prepared. Also, ask any member of your family or anyone going with you to ask questions that they have. **Make sure that all your concerns are addressed before your treatment begins.**

Knowledge is power when it comes to cancer treatment. Your questions are important to express and to be answered. Any questions or concerns can be expressed as part of caring for yourself or someone else who needs answers, whether healthcare providers, friends, family members or employers.

You may be asked at some point if you want to participate in research studies. You should ask these questions beforehand and participate in the studies only if you agree with the research procedures, test results, and other information shared with you by the research team.

You should also remember that any medical information provided by a physician or other healthcare provider is always subject to change without notice due to evolving science, medicine, clinical practice guidelines, and federal regulations.

There are no guarantees that any statement about conditions you may experience or treatments stated or recommended will remain true once treatment has been started. You should not use the information for yourself, but it is vital to provide this information to your physicians if they ask.

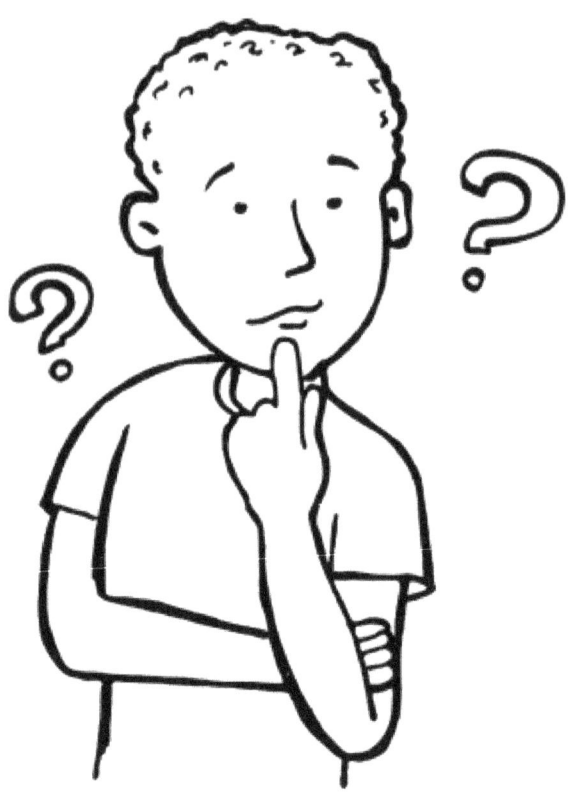

God And Chemotherapy Treatment.

How can God help me during cancer and chemotherapy treatment?

God has power and can help you during chemotherapy treatment.

Say this **prayer for strength**:

"I will stand fast in God's ability to deliver me from the tests that I am facing in life. No matter what is happening, I know that God is with me, and He can deliver me out of this situation. Only God can help me through my difficult situation and give me a way out of it. The Lord has promised me a way through this difficulty, and He will help me get over it. This is His promise. He will see me through it and give me the strength to get through every step of it.

I know that God can take away my pain, but He wants my cooperation. I have already asked Him to help me get over this problem, and He has promised to heal me. Therefore, I have decided to trust in His promise for healing and not worry about it anymore. I believe that God can deliver me from cancer treatment, even while I am receiving chemotherapy treatment.

If I do not trust in God's promise and walk on in faith, I will never come out of this trouble. I believe that God will help me through this situation, even while I am receiving chemotherapy treatment. No matter how much pain I am going through and how much sickness is attacking my body, I know that God can deliver me from it.

God has promised that He will take away the pain if only we will depend on Him alone."

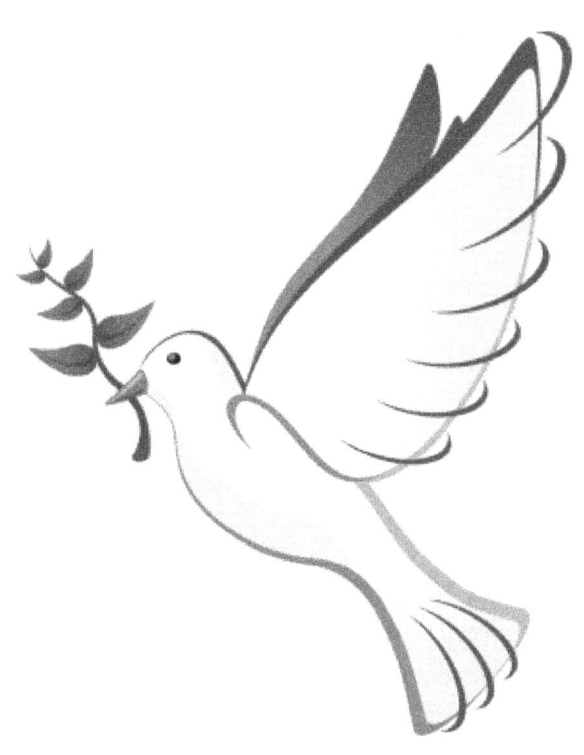

Bible Verses

Romans 8:28

And we know that all things work together for good to them that love God, to them who are the called according to his purpose.

2 Corinthians 12:7-10

And lest I should be exalted above measure through the abundance of the revelations, there was given to me a thorn in the flesh, the messenger of Satan to buffet me, lest I should be exalted above measure. For this thing, I besought the Lord thrice, that it might depart from me.

And he said unto me, My grace is sufficient for thee: for my strength is made perfect in weakness. Most gladly, therefore, will I rather glory in my infirmities, that the power of Christ may rest upon me. Therefore I take pleasure in infirmity, in reproaches, in necessities, in persecutions, in distresses for Christ's sake: for when I am weak, then am I strong.

Isaiah 41:10

Fear thou not; for I am with thee: be not dismayed; for I am thy God: I will strengthen thee; yea, I will help thee; yea, I will uphold thee with the right hand of my righteousness.

Psalm 107:19-20

And he sent darkness and made it dark, and they rebelled not against his word.

He turned their waters into blood and slew their fish.

Matthew 8:17-18

That it might be fulfilled which was spoken by Esaias the prophet, saying, Himself took our infirmities, and bare [our] sicknesses. And he was wounded for our transgressions, [he was] bruised for our iniquities: the chastisement of our peace [was] upon him; and with his stripes, we are healed.

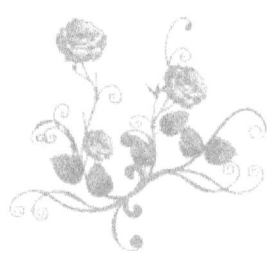

Thank you again for your purchase.

I hope you found this book valuable and helpful. If so, please give us a thumbs-up; your review is most important to assist others in their journey.

Good luck with your journey.

We are thanking you in advance.

About The Author

Anthea Peries BSc (Hons) is a published author; she completed her undergraduate studies in several sciences, including Biology, Brain and Behaviour and Child Development.

A former graduate member of the British Psychological Society, she has experience in counselling and is a former senior management executive.

Born in London, Anthea enjoys fine cuisine, writing and has travelled the world. She has a spoilt but cute but naughty black and white cat named Giorgio.

Other Books By This Author

You may be interested in other self-help books by Anthea Peries, particularly about chemotherapy cycle treatment journals, grief and bereavement, funerals, other areas such as eating disorders, food addiction, binge-eating, sugar cravings, emotional eating or, night eating syndrome, insomnia etc.

ABC's Of Salvation

Are you feeling depressed and down?

Are you seeking security?

Are you wondering what is going on in this world right now?

If you were to die tomorrow, where will your soul go, up or down?

Hell is a real place, my friend. We are not promised our last breath. We are all sinners, and the wages of sin is death. But the good news, according to Paul's Gospel, is that we can be saved right now through faith alone, not of ourselves but what Jesus Christ did on the Cross for us.

Accept his FREE gift TODAY!

Gospel = Good News

Corinthians 15:1-4

ABC OF SALVATION

A - ADMIT

Admit you are a sinner and have made mistakes.

Romans 3:23

B - BELIEVE

Believe that Jesus is God's Son, died on the Cross you, and rose from the grave on the third day.

Romans 10:9-10

C - CONFESS

Confess with your mouth that Jesus is Lord of your life. Then, commit yourself to a life of following Jesus and serving others.

Romans 10:13

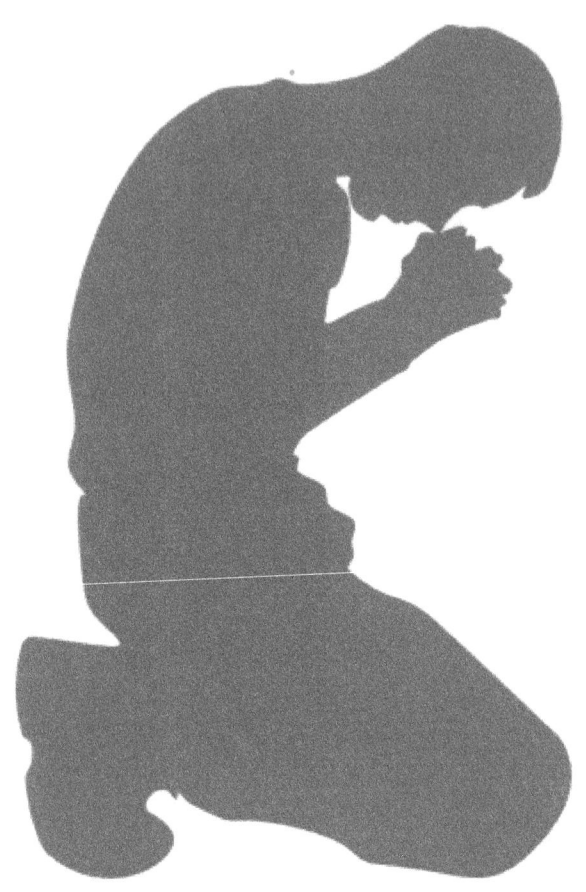

Useful Links

Top highly recommended teachers according to your style of learning:

1. Robert Breaker (Pastor/Missionary)

Website of Missionary Evangelist

https://thecloudchurch.org

Also, on YouTube

How To Get Saved: https://bit.ly/34bDBr8

Watch Robert Breaker

YouTube video (must watch!),

The Rapture of the Church:

https://tinyurl.com/TheRaptureoftheChurch

1. **Dr Andy Woods**

https://www.andywoodsministries.org/

Also, on YouTube

Listen Free Audio below:

Dr Andy Woods explains The Rapture of the Church: https://bit.ly/3vq1Fmc

1. **Pastor Gene Kim**

https://realbiblebelievers.com/about-us/pastor-gene-kim/

Also, on YouTube, Pastor Gene Kim explains dispensationalism: https://bit.ly/2RC3fTm

1. **JD Farag**

Bible Prophesy Updates, sermons and other resources:

https://www.jdfarag.org/

1. **Amir Tsarfati**

News from Israel and Bible Prophesy Updates.

https://beholdisrael.org/

https://www.youtube.com/user/beholdisrael/videos

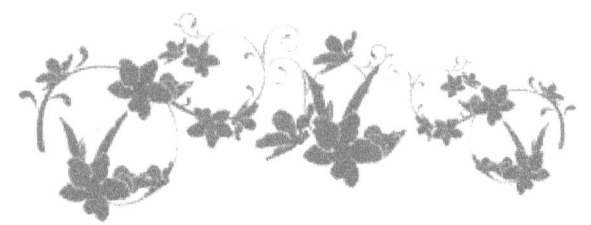

Don't miss out!

Visit the website below and you can sign up to receive emails whenever Anthea Peries publishes a new book. There's no charge and no obligation.

https://books2read.com/r/B-A-DMCG-LYVPB

BOOKS 2 READ

Connecting independent readers to independent writers.

Also by Anthea Peries

Addictions
Quit Gambling: How To Overcome Your Betting Addiction Symptoms Causes Proven Treatment Recovery
Shopping Addiction: Overcome Excessive Buying. Quit Impulse Purchasing, Save Money And Avoid Debt

Cancer and Chemotherapy
Coping with Cancer & Chemotherapy Treatment: What You Need to Know to Get Through Chemo Sessions
Coping with Cancer: How Can You Help Someone with Cancer, Dealing with Cancer Family Member, Facing Cancer Alone, Dealing with Terminal Cancer Diagnosis, Chemotherapy Treatment & Recovery
Chemotherapy Survival Guide: Coping with Cancer & Chemotherapy Treatment Side Effects
Chemotherapy Chemo Side Effects And The Holistic Approach: Alternative, Complementary And Supplementary Proven Treatments Guide For Cancer Patients

Eating Disorders
Food Cravings: Simple Strategies to Help Deal with Craving for Sugar & Junk Food
Sugar Cravings: How to Stop Sugar Addiction & Lose Weight
The Immune System, Autoimmune Diseases & Inflammatory Conditions: Improve Immunity, Eating Disorders & Eating for Health
Food Addiction: Overcome Sugar Bingeing, Overeating on Junk Food & Night Eating Syndrome
Food Addiction: Overcoming your Addiction to Sugar, Junk Food, and Binge Eating
Food Addiction: Why You Eat to Fall Asleep and How to Overcome Night Eating Syndrome
Overcome Food Addiction: How to Overcome Food Addiction, Binge Eating and Food Cravings
Healthy Gut: Transform Your Health from the Inside Out, for a Healthy You
Emotional Eating: Stop Emotional Eating & Develop Intuitive Eating Habits to Keep Your Weight Down
Emotional Eating: Overcoming Emotional Eating, Food Addiction and Binge Eating for Good
Eating At Night Time: Sleep Disorders, Health and Hunger Pangs: Tips On What You Can Do About It
Addiction To Food: Proven Help For Overcoming Binge Eating Compulsion And Dependence

Food Addiction

Overcoming Food Addiction to Sugar, Junk Food. Stop Binge Eating and Bad Emotional Eating Habits

Food Addiction: Overcoming Emotional Eating, Binge Eating and Night Eating Syndrome

Weight Loss Without Dieting: 21 Easy Ways To Lose Weight Naturally

Grief, Bereavement, Death, Loss

Coping with Loss & Dealing with Grief: Surviving Bereavement, Healing & Recovery After the Death of a Loved One

How to Plan a Funeral

Coping With Grief And Heartache Of Losing A Pet: Loss Of A Beloved Furry Companion: Easing The Pain For Those Affected By Animal Bereavement

Grieving The Loss Of Your Baby: Coping With The Devastation Shock And Heartbreak Of Losing A Child Through Miscarriage, Still Birth

Seeking Salvation, Secure In Belief: How To Get Sure-Fire Saved By Grace Through Faith, Rapture Ready And Heaven Bound

Loss And Grief: Treatment And Discovery Understanding Bereavement, Moving On From Heartbreak And Despair To Recovery

Health Fitness

How To Avoid Colds and Flu Everyday Tips to Prevent or Lessen The Impact of Viruses During Winter Season

Quark Cheese
50 More Ways to Use Quark Low-fat Soft Cheese: The Natural Alternative When Cooking Classic Meals

Quark Cheese Recipes: 21 Delicious Breakfast Smoothie Ideas Using Quark Cheese

30 Healthy Ways to Use Quark Low-fat Soft Cheese

Quit Alcohol
How To Stop Drinking Alcohol: Coping With Alcoholism, Signs, Symptoms, Proven Treatment And Recovery

Relationships
The Grief Of Getting Over A Relationship Breakup: How To Accept Breaking Up With Your Ex | Advice And Tips To Move On

Sleep Disorders
Sleep Better at Night and Cure Insomnia Especially When Stressed

Standalone

Family Style Asian Cookbook: Authentic Eurasian Recipes: Traditional Anglo-Burmese & Anglo-Indian

Coping with Loss and Dealing with Grief: The Stages of Grief and 20 Simple Ways on How to Get Through the Bad Days

Coping With Grief Of A Loved One After A Suicide: Grieving The Devastation And Loss Of Someone Who Took Their Own Life. How Long Does The Heartache Last?

When A Person Goes Missing And Cannot Be Found: Coping With The Grief And Devastation, Without Losing Hope, Of When An Adult Or Child Disappears

Menopause For Women: Signs Symptoms And Treatments A Simple Guide

Remembering Me: Discover Your Memory Proven Ways To Expand & Increase It As You Get Older

Boredom: How To Overcome Feeling Bored Discover Over 100 Proven Ways To Beat Apathy

CPSIA information can be obtained
at www.ICGtesting.com
Printed in the USA
LVHW040031251022
731424LV00003B/496